Cooking with Courage Cookbook

Tasty and Nutritious Recipes for Kids Facing Cancer.

Tommy W. Pate

TABLE OF CONTENTS

Introduction

Thank you for purchasing this book "Cooking with Courage: Tasty and Nutritious Recipes for Kids Facing Cancer." You or a loved one has probably been impacted by childhood cancer if you are reading this. Being told you have cancer may be frightening and upsetting, particularly for kids and their families. This cookbook fills that need by providing comfort, hope, and useful advice for sustaining the body and spirit through trying times.There is more to Cooking with Courage than simply a cookbook. It's a tool to assist families dealing with pediatric cancer in preparing nourishing and delectable meals that aid in their child's recovery. This cookbook's dishes were created with the special requirements and difficulties of cancer treatment in mind. They include nutritional components that support digestion, strengthen the immune system, and replenish nutrients that are often lost during therapy.

That's not all, however. Cooking with Courage acknowledges the value of food in uniting families and boosting spirits in trying times. This cookbook contains kid-friendly, enjoyable to prepare and delectable dishes. They are intended to stimulate creativity and promote family involvement in the culinary process, fostering a feeling of fun and community in the kitchen.

This cookbook also offers guidance on meal planning while receiving cancer treatment, resources for families impacted by childhood cancer, and useful tips and methods for cooking with kids. The recipes in Cooking with Courage should provide families dealing with children's cancer sustenance, pleasure, and a feeling of community during a trying time. We hope that Cooking with Courage will serve as a source of inspiration and comfort for them.

We appreciate you selecting Cooking with Courage. Let's start a meal!

(A.) <u>Introducing Childhood Cancer</u>

A diagnosis of childhood cancer is distressing for any family. Cancer that is discovered in children and young people under the age of 20 is referred to by this phrase. Over 11,050 children in the United States under the age of 15 get cancer diagnoses each year, according to the American Cancer Society.Leukemia, lymphoma, brain, and central nervous system cancers, neuroblastoma, Wilms tumors, and bone cancer are the most prevalent kinds of pediatric cancer. Although the exact causes of childhood cancer are unknown, certain illnesses, radiation exposure, exposure to particular chemicals, and genetic factors have all been associated with a higher chance of developing the disease.

(B.)<u>Identification and Therapy for Cancer</u>

Blood tests, imaging scans, and biopsies are just a few of the many tests and procedures that may be used to diagnose children's cancer. Cancer in children may be treated surgically, with radiation, chemotherapy, and immunotherapy. The sort of therapy will be determined by cancer type and stage, the child's age, and general health.

(C.) The effects of pediatric cancer

The whole family is impacted by childhood cancer, not just the kid. The course of treatment may be drawn out and difficult, often requiring repeated hospital admissions. The kid and family may experience a great deal of emotional distress, including dread, worry, and uncertainty.

(D.) Childhood Cancer and Nutrition

In order to sustain a child's health while receiving cancer treatment, nutrition is essential. A good diet may encourage healthy development, strengthen the immune system, and enhance the quality of life. Yet, a child's appetite and digestion may be affected by cancer therapy, making it difficult to maintain a nutritious diet.The dishes in this book are created with an awareness of the special requirements and difficulties associated with cancer treatment. They include nutritional components that support digestion, strengthen the immune system, and replenish nutrients that are often lost during therapy.

For any family, dealing with childhood cancer is a challenging and heartbreaking road. Families may, however, travel this path with bravery and optimism if they are provided with the necessary tools and support. It's more than simply a cookbook when it comes to Cooking with Courage: Tasty and Nutritious Recipes for Kids Facing Cancer. It is a tool to assist families dealing with children's cancer in preparing wholesome and delectable meals that will aid in their child's rehabilitation, make cooking enjoyable, and provide a feeling of community during a trying time.

(E.) Recognizing the effects of cancer on the body

Cancer is a complicated condition that may affect many bodily components. When cells in the body start to grow and divide erratically, tumors—abnormal collections of tissue—are the result. Every area of the body, including the brain, bones, organs, and blood, may be affected by cancer.

(i.)Cancer Development

Cellular DNA modifications lead to the development of cancer. Genetics, exposure to particular chemicals or radiation, and lifestyle decisions like smoking or poor eating patterns are just a few of the causes of these alterations. Tumors may develop when cells expand and divide uncontrolled due to Genetic damage.

(ii)Variety of Tumors

Tumors may be classified as benign or malignant. Noncancerous benign tumors do not metastasize to other areas of the body. They often don't develop quickly and are easily eliminated by surgery. On the other hand, malignant tumors may infect neighboring tissues and organs, spread to other areas of the body via the bloodstream or lymphatic system, and are cancerous.

(III)Cancer's effects on the body

Depending on the kind, stage, and location of the tumor, the consequences of cancer on the body might differ. Cancer may have a variety of physical effects, including:

- Immune system deterioration: Cancer cells may make it harder for the body to fend off infections and illnesses by weakening the immune system.
- Damage to neighboring tissues and organs: When cancer cells multiply and spread, they may cause harm to those tissues and organs. This may result in a range of symptoms, including pain, inflammation, and organ malfunction.
- Malnutrition: Cancer cells may deplete the body's supply of vital nutrients, resulting in undernutrition and weight loss.Cancer may contribute to weariness, which can make it difficult to carry out regular tasks.

Apart from the physical repercussions, cancer may also have psychological ones, such as stress, worry, and depression.

(F.) Nutrition's Role in Cancer Therapy

For cancer patients, a healthy diet is crucial. A nutritious diet may strengthen the immune system, promote healing, and help you stay strong and energetic. Nonetheless, a person's appetite and digestion may be affected by cancer therapy, making it challenging to maintain a nutritious diet.We put a lot of emphasis on utilizing nutritious foods to assist the body throughout cancer treatment in Cooking with Courage: Tasty and Nutritious Recipes for Kids Facing Cancer. Our recipes are made with components that support a healthy immune system, promote digestion, and replenish vital nutrients that are often lost during cancer treatments. They are created with the specific requirements and difficulties of cancer therapy in mind.Cancer is a complicated condition that may have a big impact on the body. Individuals and families affected by cancer may traverse this difficult road with bravery and hope if they understand the effects of cancer on the body and the significance of healthy nutrition throughout cancer treatment. Cooking with Courage: Tasty and Nutritious Recipes for Kids Facing Cancer may improve the health and wellness of people impacted by pediatric cancer by using nutritious ingredients and healthful dishes.

(G.) Common cancer therapies for children

Since juvenile cancer is a difficult condition, a thorough treatment strategy is necessary. Depending on the kind of cancer, its stage, and the child's general health, several treatment options may be available. The following are some of the most typical cancer therapies for kids:

1.)Surgery: For many forms of pediatric malignancies, surgery is often the initial course of therapy. Surgery aims to remove as much of the tumor as feasible while causing the least amount of harm to healthy tissue. Surgery could be followed by further therapies including radiation therapy or chemotherapy, depending on the location and size of the tumor.

2.)Chemotherapy: it employs chemicals to destroy cancer cells throughout the body as a systemic treatment. Chemotherapy often coexists with other therapies like surgery or radiation therapy. Chemotherapy may be administered orally, intravenously, or intravenously into the tumor.

3.)High-energy radiation: This is used in radiation treatment to eliminate cancer cells. Before or after surgery, it is often used to reduce tumor size or to eradicate any cancer cells that may have survived. Moreover, radiation treatment and chemotherapy may be used together.

4.)A bone marrow transplant: it is commonly referred to as a stem cell transplant involves replacing diseased or destroyed bone marrow with healthy stem cells. You may either get stem cells from a donor or from your own body.

5.)Immunotherapy: An approach to treating cancer that makes use of the immune system of the patient's body. This may be accomplished either by improving the immune system's capacity to identify and combat cancer cells or by utilizing modified immune cells that specifically target cancer cells.

6.)Targeted therapy: is a form of medicine that specifically targets certain molecules or proteins in cancer cells. This may lessen the harm done to healthy cells while aiding in the slowing or stopping of the development of cancer cells.

These therapies may be successful in treating pediatric cancer, but they also carry a risk of negative side effects. An immune system that is compromised, exhaustion, nausea, vomiting, and hair loss are typical side effects of cancer therapy. Controlling side effects is a crucial component of cancer therapy, and medical professionals will collaborate with patients and their families to create an all-inclusive care plan that takes into account all facets of cancer treatment and recovery.

We recognize the value of providing the body with nutrition while undergoing cancer treatment in Cooking with Courage: Tasty and Nutritious Recipes for Kids Facing Cancer. Our dishes are created to be quick and simple to make, packed with nutrients, and tasty, giving people and families the energy they need to sustain their bodies during cancer treatment. We can support the health and wellness of people impacted by pediatric cancer by collaborating with healthcare professionals.

Chapter 1

How proper nutrition may aid in the treatment and recovery from cancer

Good nutrition is essential for these processes. Eating a balanced diet helps strengthen the immune system, reduces the negative effects of cancer therapy, and provides the body with the resources it needs to fight cancer.The body needs more calories and nutrients during cancer therapy than it does at other times. This is due to the fact that cancer treatment side effects including nausea, vomiting, and diarrhea may make it challenging for patients to consume adequate food. Moreover, the body may use more energy during cancer therapy than usual, necessitating higher calorie intake to maintain weight.

Eating a balanced, nutrient-rich diet is crucial to supporting cancer treatment and recovery. Consuming a range of fruits, vegetables, whole grains, lean protein, and healthy fats is necessary to achieve this. Drinking lots of water and other drinks can help you remain hydrated.

Some particular nutrients that are crucial for those receiving cancer therapy include:

- Protein: The creation and repair of bodily tissues depend on protein. It is particularly crucial during cancer treatment since it may guard against muscle wasting and strengthen the immune system.

- Eating sufficient calories is crucial for weight maintenance and for giving the body the energy it needs to fight cancer. It might be difficult to maintain this throughout cancer treatment, so it's crucial to choose meals that are rich in calories and nutritional density.

- Minerals and vitamins: Minerals and vitamins are crucial for boosting the immune system and general health. In order to make sure that the body is receiving all the nutrients it needs, it is crucial to consume a variety of fruits and vegetables.

- Fiber: Fiber is crucial for supporting digestive health and reducing constipation, which is often a side effect of cancer therapy.

A proper diet may aid in lowering the risk of cancer recurrence in addition to aiding cancer therapy and recovery. Inflammation in the body, which is a recognized risk factor for cancer, may be reduced by eating a nutritious diet that is rich in fruits, vegetables, and whole grains.

Many foods and minerals may have anti-cancer capabilities, according to research. For instance, according to some research, cruciferous vegetables like broccoli and cauliflower may cut the risk of cancer by facilitating the body's removal of cancer-causing chemicals. According to other research, antioxidant-rich foods like berries and leafy greens may aid to reduce DNA damage, which may result in cancer.

It is crucial to remember that although a good diet may aid in the treatment and prevention of cancer, it cannot take the place of medical care. Cancer patients should collaborate closely with their medical professionals to create a thorough care plan that covers all areas of their recovery and treatment. We are dedicated to giving people and families the information and resources they need in this book to assist their health and well-being while undergoing cancer treatment. Our cookbook offers nourishing and delectable dishes that are simple to create at home in an effort to make mealtime simpler and more fun for families dealing with pediatric cancer. Focusing on providing the body with wholesome nutrients may improve cancer treatment and recovery while also advancing general health and well-being..

Cooking with Kids

Cooking with children is a fun and interesting approach to teaching them valuable life skills and getting them interested in developing good eating habits. Early cooking instruction increases a child's likelihood of making good food choices throughout their life and of having a positive connection with food.

Cooking with children offers a wealth of chances for development and learning. Youngsters may pick up knowledge about various ingredients, cooking methods, and kitchen safety. Kids may also learn crucial abilities like measuring items, reading and following recipes, and cooperating with others.While cooking with children, it's crucial to choose recipes that are suitable for their ages and to keep an eye on them at all times. Although older kids may do more difficult chores like planning meals and creating recipes, younger kids may require assistance with simple tasks like chopping and using the stove.

Children's participation and interest in eating may be increased by including them in the planning and preparation of meals. Children might feel more immersed in the dinner and improve their decision-making abilities by being encouraged to select recipes and assist with food shopping.

For families dealing with pediatric cancer, cooking with children might be very useful. Children may find it challenging to eat as a result of a variety of side effects from cancer treatment, so including them in the planning and preparation of meals may make mealtimes more interesting and fun. Also, while many areas of life may seem unexpected and out of control, cooking with children may help establish a sense of rhythm and normality.

Children's development of critical social and emotional skills may also benefit from cooking. Cooking with friends teaches kids how to speak clearly, cooperate with others, and function as a team. While kids attempt to solve problems that could emerge while cooking, they also acquire crucial problem-solving abilities. Children's confidence and a healthy sense of self may both be fostered by cooking with them. Children may grow a feeling of pride and success when they take on new chores in the kitchen and see the results of their effort. This may boost their self-confidence and self-esteem and promote a lifetime love of cooking and nutritious eating.

At a trying moment, families may foster a feeling of closeness and community by cooking together. Parents may boost their child's health and wellness by feeding them wholesome meals.

With the aid of this book, families may experience the fun of cooking with children and promote their child's well-being and health while undergoing pediatric cancer treatment.

Advice for cooking with kids

Cooking with kids may be enjoyable and rewarding, but it can also be difficult at times. The following advice can help you have a more positive and successful experience:

- Choose dishes that are suitable for your child's age: Choose recipes that are suitable for your child's age and degree of expertise. Older kids may be able to manage more complicated dishes, while younger kids could require basic recipes with fewer steps.
- In advance: Gather all the required supplies and tools and read the recipe before you start. The cooking procedure will become easier and more effective as a result.
- Offer age-appropriate chores: Older children can manage more sophisticated

jobs like slicing vegetables and managing the stove, while smaller children can be given basic duties like stirring, measuring materials, and adding toppings.

- Educate your kid about kitchen safety. Make sure they are aware of fundamental guidelines like washing their hands before handling food, putting on oven gloves when handling hot objects, and never leaving the stove unattended.
- Funnel it out: Encourage your youngster to use their imagination while cooking and to try new tastes and ingredients. To make the process more entertaining, use amusing kitchenware and equipment like colored mixing bowls and cookie cutters.Stressing healthy options can help your kid learn about good eating practices and expose them to new fruits, veggies, and whole grains.
- Be patient: Cooking with kids may be messy and time-consuming; as a result, be patient and give the procedure plenty of time.

You can make cooking with kids enjoyable and interesting for the entire family by using the advice in this article. And keep in mind that having fun and enjoying your time cooking together is what matters most!.

Age-Appropriate Cooking Chores

To guarantee children's safety and success in the kitchen, assign age-appropriate tasks while cooking with them. According to age, below are some recommendations for culinary tasks:

- Years 2-3: Youngsters in this age range may assist with basic activities including washing produce, tearing lettuce, and combining ingredients. Also, they may assist with the cupcake and cookie decorating.
- Years 4-5: At this age, kids may start assisting with tasks like measuring materials, using cookie cutters, and stirring ingredients. Also, they may assist with meal preparation and cleanup.

- Years 6-7: Kids in this age range may begin to do more difficult chores including breaking eggs, peeling vegetables, and using a whisk. Using a plastic knife, they may also assist in slicing delicate fruits and veggies.
- Years 8 to 9: Under the supervision of an adult, kids may start using a standard knife to chop fruits and vegetables at this age. Also, they may assist with putting together sandwiches, blending smoothies, and following basic instructions.
- Ages 10 to 12: Kids in this age range are capable of more difficult chores like scrambling eggs and sautéing vegetables. They can even make basic dishes on their own. They can also assist with making shopping lists and food planning.

It's crucial to keep in mind that every youngster is unique and may have varying degrees of cooking proficiency. Children should always be supervised while using knives or hot appliances, and you should always go through kitchen safety precautions with them. While cooking with kids, giving them age-appropriate responsibilities may help them become more self-assured and adept in the kitchen while also teaching them valuable life lessons like meal planning, a nutritious diet, and kitchen safety. Children may desire to undertake increasingly difficult culinary activities as they gain expertise in the kitchen. More suggestions for culinary activities suitable for older kids and teens are provided below:

- 13–15 years old: At this age, kids may start experimenting with more complicated recipes and methods, such as making their own pasta, baking bread, or using a food processor or blender. Also, they may start studying fundamental culinary methods like grilling and roasting.
- Teens may take on greater responsibility in the kitchen and may be motivated to learn how to make meals for the whole family when they reach the age of 16 to 18. Also, they may begin creating their own recipes and experimenting with

various tastes and ingredients. Also, they may pick up more sophisticated culinary methods including braising, poaching, and smoking.

In encouraging youngsters to embark on challenging projects, it's crucial, to be honest with them about their capabilities. Never leave kids alone in the kitchen and always provide instruction and supervision as required.
Cooking with children is a wonderful way to spend time as a family and teach them valuable life lessons. Children may acquire a passion for cooking that will benefit them throughout their lives by assigning age-appropriate chores and offering direction and assistance.

Chapter 2

Having kids enjoy and be interested in cooking

Children of all ages may enjoy cooking, but some youngsters who feel scared or overpowered in the kitchen may find it to be a difficult chore. Here are some ideas for engaging and entertaining youngsters in the kitchen:

A.)Choose recipes that are entertaining and participatory, with plenty of hands-on activities and enticing visuals. Kids may have a lot of fun in the kitchen by helping with recipes that call for rolling out dough, using cookie cutters to cut out designs, or decorating cookies or cupcakes.

B.)Make it a game: Create challenges or contests to make cooking into a game. Children may be challenged to cook the quickest pizza or the most vibrant salad, for instance.

C.)Employ entertaining and eye-catching kitchenware: Using entertaining and eye-catching kitchenware may make cooking for youngsters more enjoyable and interesting. Spatulas, whisks, and measuring cups are just a few of the kitchen tools that are suitable for children.

D.)Encourage youngsters to explore new tastes and textures by being creative with the items they use. Asking children to recommend their preferred ingredients or recipes is another way to include them in the meal preparation process.

E.)Make cooking a sensory experience for children by having them smell, touch, and taste the ingredients. Their taste awareness and palate development may benefit from this.

F.)Let kids be in charge: Giving kids the reins in the kitchen may boost their self-esteem and feeling of independence. Give them projects that are suitable for their age and, when required, provide direction and help.

G.)Make it a social activity: Cooking with loved ones and friends may be a wonderful way to spend time together. Include children in the process of selecting and preparing meals, and encourage them to invite their friends over for an entertaining and educational cooking party.

You can encourage children to develop a love of cooking and healthy eating habits that will benefit them throughout their life by making cooking enjoyable and interesting for them. With the help of these suggestions, teaching kids to cook can be a productive and enjoyable experience for everyone.

Breakfast to Eat and Their Preparation

Breakfast is a crucial portion of a child's day, and it's vital to feed them the correct nutrients to provide them the energy they need to battle cancer.The following are some breakfast suggestions for children with cancer;

- Berry Oatmeal: Due to its high fiber content and simple digestion, oatmeal is a fantastic breakfast choice for children with cancer. For more taste and nutrients, mix in some fruit like strawberries, blueberries, or raspberries with the oats.

- Smoothies for breakfast are a great way to include a lot of nutrients in a delectable and convenient meal. To prepare a smooth and delectable smoothie, blend some fruits like bananas, mangoes, and berries with some milk or yogurt.
- Bread with peanut butter and bananas is a delicious way to get some protein, fiber, and potassium into your diet. For a quick and simple breakfast, spread some peanut butter on whole-wheat bread and top it with banana slices.
- Egg Muffins: Including some protein in your child's breakfast with egg muffins is a terrific idea. For a quick and wholesome meal that can be had on the go, combine some eggs, cheese, and vegetables like spinach or mushrooms. Bake the mixture in a muffin pan.
- Pancakes and waffles: By using whole-grain flour and using fruit like blueberries or sliced bananas, pancakes and waffles may be made healthier. These can be a fun and decadent morning

alternative. To add more protein, top them with some Greek yogurt or peanut butter.

- It's crucial to concentrate on nutrient-dense, easily digestible foods when developing breakfast meals for children. Proper nutrition can assist a child's immune system and provide them with the energy they need to battle cancer.

Also, getting kids involved in the preparation of breakfast may turn it into a pleasant activity that will motivate them to have a nutritious breakfast every day.For families that may have a hectic schedule owing to cancer treatment appointments and other activities, including breakfast foods that are simple to make and can be eaten on the go might be very beneficial. Provide a range of tastes and textures to keep things interesting while creating breakfast dishes for children with cancer. This may guard against food boredom and guarantee that kids are consuming a variety of nutrients from various meals.

As an example, adding nuts and seeds to oatmeal or smoothies may offer protein, healthy fats, and crunch. In addition to adding a warm, comforting taste to pancakes and waffles, adding spices like cinnamon or nutmeg also has health advantages including lowering inflammation. Also, it's crucial to consider any dietary preferences or limitations that kids with cancer could have. Provide bland, low-fat breakfast alternatives like bread or crackers to a kid who is suffering nausea or vomiting as a side effect of chemotherapy, for instance.

In conclusion, giving breakfast alternatives that are scrumptious and nourishing to children with cancer may be an important part of their overall treatment strategy. This book may provide families with quick and wholesome breakfast alternatives that can aid in their child's recovery and general well-being by integrating a range of tastes and textures as well as taking dietary restrictions and preferences into account.

<u>Nutritious breakfast recipes to start the day off right</u>

Everyone should have a healthy breakfast, but children with cancer need it even more because they must fuel their bodies for the arduous struggle that lies ahead. Giving them a nutritious and nourishing breakfast may boost their appetite, strengthen their immune systems, and give them the energy they need to battle cancer. For children with cancer, try these wholesome breakfast dishes to get their day off to a good start:

1.)Avocado Toast: Packed with fiber, vitamins, and healthy fats, avocado toast is a simple but tasty breakfast option. Sliced tomatoes, salt, and pepper, along with avocado are added to whole-grain bread after it has been mashed. Poached eggs may be added on top for more protein.

2.)Yogurt Parfait: Eating a variety of healthy items in a yogurt parfait is entertaining and simple. For a vibrant and filling breakfast, combine Greek yogurt, mixed berries, oats, and honey in a glass or jar.

3.)Quinoa breakfast bowl: Quinoa is rich in fiber and antioxidants and is a complete protein. Add your preferred toppings, such as sliced bananas, berries, almonds, and seeds, after cooking the quinoa with milk and cinnamon.

4.)Smoothie bowl for breakfast: A smoothie bowl is a thicker smoothie that can be eaten with a spoon. Greek yogurt, milk, honey, and frozen fruit are blended; sliced fruit, granola, and nuts are then sprinkled on top for taste and texture.

5.)Banana Oat Pancakes: By using whole-grain flour and using oats for fiber and nutrients, pancakes may be made healthier. To prepare pancake batter, mash a ripe banana and combine it with oats, eggs, and milk. Sliced bananas and maple syrup are placed on top while cooking on a nonstick pan.

6.)Scrambled eggs with veggies are a delicious way to boost the nutritional value of your breakfast. Spinach, mushrooms, and peppers are sauteed before eggs are added and scrambled until done. Serve with whole-grain bread for a balanced meal.While cooking healthy breakfasts for kids with cancer, it is vital to emphasize whole foods that are rich in nutrients and simple to digest. Also, getting kids involved in the preparation of breakfast may turn it into a pleasant activity that will motivate them to have a nutritious breakfast every day. Cooking with Courage can improve the health and recovery of children with cancer by offering nutritious and delectable breakfast alternatives.

Vitamins and Minerals-rich juices and Smoothies for Breakfast

Morning juices and smoothies may be a great way for children with cancer to get a lot of nutrients in one meal. These beverages may provide a variety of vitamins, minerals, and antioxidants to strengthen a person's immune system, assist with digestion, and fight cancer when made with the proper components. Here are some suggestions for vitamin and mineral-rich morning juices and smoothies for children with cancer:

- Green smoothies are a great way to receive a range of nutrients in one serving. Combine spinach, kale, avocado, banana, and coconut milk in a blender to make a creamy, delectable beverage that is also vitamin and mineral-rich.

- Smoothie with berries: Berries are a fantastic source of fiber and are high in antioxidants. For a healthy and energizing smoothie, combine milk, Greek yogurt, honey, and mixed berries.

- Juice made from carrots and apples: Vitamin C-rich carrots and apples may help strengthen the immune system. Combine carrots, apples, and ginger in a juicer to create a nutrient-rich beverage that is sweet and tangy.

- Mango, pineapple, and papaya are among the tropical fruits that are high in vitamin C and other nutrients. For a tasty and cool smoothie, combine frozen tropical fruits, coconut milk, and Greek yogurt.

- Beet Juice: Beets are rich in antioxidants and may assist maintain liver function. For a colorful and nourishing beverage, combine beets, carrots, apples, and ginger in the juicer.
- Chocolate Banana Smoothie: For a richer breakfast alternative, combine frozen bananas with almond milk, cocoa powder, honey, and other ingredients to create a decadent but wholesome chocolate smoothie.

It's crucial to use whole, fresh ingredients and stay away from added sugars or artificial sweeteners when preparing morning smoothies and juices for children with cancer. Juices and smoothies may keep kids hydrated and fed while they are receiving cancer treatment and can be a fun way to expose them to new fruits and veggies. Cooking with Courage may promote the health and well-being of kids with cancer by offering delicious and nutrient-rich breakfast alternatives.

Breakfast items to pack in a hurry for a busy morning

Mornings may be a difficult time, particularly for families with a child undergoing cancer treatment. Having quick and simple portable breakfast alternatives might help make hectic mornings a bit less stressful. Here are some suggestions for portable meals that are filling and practical:

- Overnight oats are a quick and filling breakfast alternative that can be made the night before and kept in a travel-friendly container. Just combine milk or yogurt, rolled oats, and your preferred additions of fruit, nuts, or seeds in a container and chill overnight.

- Breakfast wraps A flexible and portable choice, breakfast wraps may be tailored to a variety of preferences. Put scrambled eggs, cheese, veggies, and lean proteins like turkey or chicken into whole-grain tortillas or wraps.

- Energy Bites: You may prepare energy bites ahead of time and put them in the refrigerator for a convenient breakfast on the go. Roll the mixture into balls, add your favorite mix-ins, such as chocolate chips or dried fruit, like peanut butter and honey, and then store in an airtight container.

- Yogurt Parfait: Yogurt parfaits may be created using yogurt, granola, and fruit as an easy and portable breakfast alternative. When you're ready to dine, layer the ingredients in a carry-on container and refrigerate.

- Fruit and Nut Butter: A quick and wholesome breakfast that can be had on the fly is fruit and nut butter. For a quick and filling breakfast, spread nut butter over a banana, an apple, or a rice cake.

- Breakfast Muffins: Breakfast muffins may be baked ahead of time and kept in the refrigerator or freezer for a quick breakfast choice. Utilize whole-grain flour and add fruits, vegetables, nuts, and seeds to boost the nutritious richness of the muffins.

Cooking with Courage may assist busy families in making sure that their kid is getting the nutrition they need while receiving cancer treatment by offering portable and nourishing breakfast alternatives. These breakfast options may be prepared ahead of time, making hectic mornings a bit simpler and less stressful.

Chapter 3

Snacks and Small Bites

A kid with cancer may need to include snacks and tiny nibbles in their meals on a regular basis. A child's appetite and taste buds may be affected by cancer treatments including chemotherapy, radiation therapy, and surgery, making it difficult for them to consume regular meals. Snacks and quick meals may provide cancer-stricken kids with the nourishment and energy they need to battle the illness and deal with its adverse effects.Planning snacks and tiny nibbles for kids with cancer requires taking their nutritional requirements into account. The construction and repair of tissues depend on protein and good fats, whereas energy comes from carbs. During undergoing cancer therapy, fiber might be particularly crucial for maintaining gut health. Other essential sources of vitamins and minerals that assist the immune system are fresh fruits and vegetables.

Snacks and small meals like the following may be helpful for children with cancer.

1.)Smoothies: Smoothies are a fantastic method to consume both calories and nutrients. A variety of fruits and vegetables, yogurt or milk, and protein powder may all be used to make them. Consider alternatives like strawberries, blueberries, almond milk, and chia seeds or spinach, banana, peanut butter, and Greek yogurt.

2.)Cheese and crackers: A traditional snack that may be tailored to the child's tastes is cheese and crackers. Cheese is a rich source of calcium and protein, while whole-grain crackers are a wonderful source of fiber.

3.)Trail mix is a portable, healthy snack that may be customized to a child's preferences. Healthy fats, protein, and fiber may be found in a combination of nuts, seeds, and dried fruits.

4.)Hummus with vegetables: Hummus is a delectable and nutritious dip that goes well with a wide range of vegetables, including carrots, celery, and cucumber. The veggies provide vitamins and minerals, while the hummus is high in protein, fiber, and healthy fats.

5.)Yogurt parfaits are tasty and wholesome snacks that may be tailored to a child's tastes. Although fresh fruit offers vitamins and fiber, Greek yogurt offers calcium and protein. For a crunchier texture, granola may also be used.

6.)Fruit and nuts: For a fast and simple snack, combine nuts, such as peanut or almond butter, with sliced apples, bananas, or other fruits. Although nut butter offers protein and good fats, fruit offers vitamins and fiber.

7.)Eggs, either hard-boiled or soft-boiled, are a fantastic source of protein and go well with whole-grain crackers.

Avoiding items that may be difficult to digest or that may irritate the digestive system is vital when preparing snacks and tiny nibbles for children with cancer. Fried or spicy meals, carbonated beverages, and highly processed snacks with added sugars are a few items to stay away from.

It's crucial to consider a child's treatment schedule while preparing snacks and small meals for them if they have cancer. Children may have nausea, vomiting, or mouth sores, which may make it difficult for them to eat or tolerate particular meals, depending on the kind of medication and the adverse effects.

For instance, offering soft, cold, or lukewarm meals like smoothies, yogurt, or mashed potatoes to a kid who has mouth sores may be beneficial. Avoiding meals that are acidic or spicy until the sores have healed can help prevent irritation and pain.

Also, the child's unique tastes and hunger should be taken into account. Throughout cancer treatment, children's tastes may alter, and they may find that things they previously liked no longer appeal to them. Offering a range of meals and tastes is crucial, as is encouraging the youngster to try new things. Providing little snacks often during the day may also be beneficial since some kids may find it simpler to consume smaller servings.

Snacks and quick meals may provide children with cancer comfort and delight in addition to providing nutrients and energy. Offering the kid their preferred snack or treat, for instance, might uplift their spirits and make them feel more normal during trying times.

Finally, it's important to include the kid as much as you can in the preparation of snacks and little bites. When a youngster feels like they have little influence over their health, letting them pick their snacks or assist with preparation may offer them a feeling of control and autonomy.

In conclusion, snacks and little nibbles may be a vital part of a child with cancer's diet, giving them comfort and pleasure in addition to vital nutrients and energy. Parents and caregivers may support a child's general health and well-being while they are receiving cancer treatment by taking into account the child's dietary requirements, treatment schedule, and personal preferences, and involving them in the process.

Healthy snacks may be an excellent way to fill the gap between meals and provide the body with the energy and nutrition it needs for peak physical and mental performance. Snacks may delay hunger, speed up metabolism, and keep blood sugar levels stable all day.

The nutritional density of the snack you choose should be taken into account. Foods that are rich in nutrients provide a lot of vitamins, minerals, and other healthy substances for not many calories. This may support satiety and provide the body with the resources and energy it needs to perform at its best.

Here are some examples of nutritious between-meal snacks:

- Fresh fruit: A terrific choice for a nutritious snack, fresh fruit is a great source of vitamins, minerals, and fiber. During the day, apples, bananas, berries, and grapes are all convenient and portable snacks.

- Vegetables with hummus: A fantastic approach to obtain a mix of fiber, protein, and healthy fats is to consume raw veggies such as carrots, celery, cucumbers, and bell peppers with hummus. A high supply of vitamins and minerals is also found in hummus.

- Nuts and seeds: Nuts and seeds are a fantastic source of protein, fiber, and good fats. For a nutritious snack, consider pumpkin seeds, cashews, almonds, and walnuts.

- Berries with Greek yogurt: Berries provide antioxidants and fiber, while Greek yogurt is a fantastic source of protein and calcium. A sprinkling of nuts or seeds may also offer more beneficial fats.

- Eggs, whether hard-boiled or soft-boiled, are a wonderful source of protein and go well with whole-grain crackers or vegetables.

- Cheese with whole-grain crackers: Cheese is a rich source of calcium and protein, while whole-grain crackers provide fiber. For a healthy snack, use low-fat cheese varieties.
- Edamame: Edamame may be eaten as a snack or added to salads and stir-fries. It is a fantastic source of protein and fiber.
- Smoothies: They're a terrific method to get both calories and nutrients. A variety of fruits, vegetables, yogurt or milk, and protein powder may be used to make them.

Avoid processed meals and snacks that are heavy in added sugars, saturated and trans fats, and salt when selecting snacks. These kinds of snacks may increase the risk of developing chronic conditions including type 2 diabetes, heart disease, and obesity.

In conclusion, nutritious snacks may provide the body with the nutrition and energy it needs to maintain physical and mental function in between meals. People may maintain good health and stave off chronic illnesses by selecting nutrient-dense meals like Greek yogurt, fresh fruits and vegetables, nuts, and seeds. When feasible, choose whole, natural foods over manufactured snacks that are heavy in harmful fats and added sugars.

It's not only about the food's nutritional content when it comes to snacks for children with cancer. Here are some suggestions for entertaining and inventive snack presentations. Snacks may be made to seem more enticing and pleasurable by using presentation. Children with cancer might benefit from cheery and imaginative food displays that make snack time more fun.For kids with cancer, here are some suggestions for entertaining and inventive food presentations:

- Fruit skewers: Snack time may be made more enjoyable and appetizing by skewering a variety of vibrant fruits including strawberries, kiwis, and pineapple. Honey or a yogurt dip may also be used to enhance the taste of the snack.

- Vegetable cups: In tiny plastic cups, layer hummus or dip with bright vegetables like carrots, celery, and cherry tomatoes. The colorful presentation makes it more enticing, and the cups make it simple for kids to take and go.
- Fruit and animal crackers: Arrange fruit slices on a platter with animal crackers to represent the background. Use blueberries to make a pond and bananas to make trees, for instance.
- Ants on a log: By adopting innovative presentation techniques, simple treats like ants on a log may be made more entertaining. Use celery sticks as the log and cream cheese or peanut butter as the "filling." Add raisins on the top to make "ants."
- Whole wheat English muffins may be used as the crust for mini-pizzas. Add cheese, tomato sauce, and toppings like

ham or turkey, or vegetables. Cut them into interesting designs like stars or hearts.

- Create fruit creatures with toothpicks and little bits of fruit. For instance, to make a tasty and nutritious snack, use a piece of banana for the body, strawberries for the ears, and blueberries for the eyes.
- Trail mix: To make a great trail mix, blend a variety of nuts, seeds, and dried fruit. Make it simple for kids to grab and go by using little bags or containers.
- Sandwich forms: Cut out colorful shapes from whole-grain bread using cookie cutters, then fill with hummus and vegetables, ham and cheese, or peanut butter and jelly.

It's crucial to take into account any dietary limitations or allergies the youngster may have while coming up with entertaining and imaginative snack presentations. Include the youngster in the process by letting them choose their own food or assist with the presentation. While they may feel like they have little influence over their health, this might offer them a feeling of control and empowerment.

In conclusion, entertaining and imaginative food displays may make snack time more pleasurable for kids with cancer. Parents and other adults who are responsible for children may make snack time more enjoyable and empowering by using bright fruits and vegetables, arranging food in amusing shapes, and including the kid in the process.

Easy dishes that children may prepare on their own

For children with cancer, cooking can be an enjoyable and empowering hobby since it gives them control over their dietary choices and a feeling of success. Yet, it's crucial to choose straightforward recipes that kids can prepare alone, without requiring a lot of supervision or help.

Children with cancer may prepare the following simple dishes on their own:

- Put some peanut butter on a tortilla, top it with some sliced banana, then wrap it up. For a tasty snack, cut the roll-up into bite-sized pieces.
- Trail Mix: In a dish, combine different nuts, seeds, and dried fruit. Youngsters may personalize their trail mix by selecting the items they choose.
- Smoothie: For a tasty and nourishing smoothie, combine a banana, frozen berries, yogurt, and a dash of milk. Children may play around with various fruits and additives to develop their own smoothie concoctions.
- Toast a piece of bread, then put mashed avocado on top for avocado toast. Add some salt and pepper, as well as various garnishes like tomato slices or cooked eggs.
- Fruit salad: Slice up a variety of fruit, including strawberries, kiwis, and pineapple, then combine the pieces in a

dish. For added taste, kids may pour some yogurt or honey.

- Butter two pieces of bread, sandwiching cheese between them to make a grilled cheese sandwich. Fry in a frying pan until the bread is crispy and the cheese is melted.
- Layer yogurt, and granola, and cut fruit in a glass or dish to make a parfait. Kids may design their own parfait by selecting the yogurt and toppings that they want.

It's crucial to check that all items are suitable for the dietary requirements and sensitivities of cancer-stricken youngsters while cooking with them. Also, it's essential to provide sufficient oversight and direction as required to guarantee their safety in the kitchen.

In conclusion, there are several straightforward dishes that children with cancer may prepare on their own, giving them a joyful and empowering activity while also ensuring they get the right nourishment. Parents and caregivers may empower children with cancer to take charge of their nutritional needs by selecting simple-to-make dishes that are safe and suitable for their dietary requirements.

Chapter 4

Soups and Stews

For children with cancer, soups, and stews may be excellent choices since they are simple to digest and can provide vital nutrients and moisture. Here are a few soups and stews that are filling and simple to make:

1.)Chicken noodle soup is a well-known soup that provides both veggies and protein. To make, cook celery, carrots, and chopped onions in a saucepan until they are soft. Add cooked chicken and egg noodles after bringing the chicken broth to a boil. Once the noodles are cooked through, simmer.

2.)Soup made from lentils is a fantastic source of iron, fiber, and protein. To make, cook celery, carrots, and chopped onions in a saucepan until they are soft. Add chopped tomatoes, chicken broth, and lentils. When the lentils are ready, simmer them after bringing them to a boil.

3.)Tomato Soup: Tomatoes are an excellent source of antioxidants and vitamin C. To get ready, cook chopped onions in a saucepan until they are soft. Chicken broth, canned tomatoes, and spices like basil and oregano should all be added. Once the tomatoes are soft, bring them to a boil and then simmer. Using an immersion blender, puree the soup until it is smooth.

4.)Vegetable stew: For children with cancer, vegetables including carrots, potatoes, and green beans may provide vital nutrients. To get ready, cook chopped onions in a saucepan until they are soft. Chicken stock, chopped veggies, and spices like thyme and rosemary should all be added. Bring to a boil and cook the veggies for the desired amount of time.

5.)Butternut Squash Soup: Fiber and vitamin A are both abundant in butternut squash. Butternut squash cubes should be roasted in the oven until they are soft. In a saucepan, cook chopped onions until they are soft, then add the roasted butternut squash and chicken stock. Use an immersion blender to combine until smooth.

It's crucial to make sure that all components in soups and stews for children with cancer are secure and suitable for their dietary requirements and sensitivities. Also, it's critical to check that the stews and soups are properly prepared and simple to consume. Soups and stews may be pureed until smooth if the kid has trouble swallowing or has a sore mouth to make them simpler to consume.

Bulk-preparable recipes that may be kept for later use include:

- Having simple-to-make meals and snacks on hand that can be saved for later use might be beneficial while a kid is receiving cancer treatment. The following recipes may be prepared in large quantities and frozen for later use:
- Meatballs: Meatballs may be a fantastic source of protein and are terrific in several recipes, such as meatball sandwiches or spaghetti and meatballs. To prepare, combine breadcrumbs, egg, and spices

like garlic powder and onion powder with ground beef or turkey. Create balls, then bake them in the oven. After chilling, place in a freezer bag or airtight container.

- Vegetable burgers: A delicious and wholesome substitute for hamburgers are veggie burgers. Cooked quinoa or brown rice should be combined with mashed beans, chopped vegetables like carrots and mushrooms, and spices like cumin and chili pepper while preparing. Make patties, then bake or grill them. After chilling, place in a freezer bag or airtight container.

- Muffins: For children with cancer, muffins make a fantastic grab-and-go snack. To prepare, combine the dry ingredients (flour, baking soda, sugar, etc.) in one bowl, and the wet ones (eggs, milk, oil) in another bowl. Mix the two recipes and stir with extras like blueberries or chocolate chips. After cooling, store baked goods in an airtight container or freezer bag.

- Chili: Chili may be a filling and healthy dish that is simple to reheat. To prepare, cook onions and garlic until they are soft in a saucepan. Beans, tomatoes in cans, ground beef or turkey, and spices like cumin and chili powder are also good additions. Simmer for a while to let the flavors mingle. After chilling, place in a freezer bag or airtight container.
- Chicken Casserole: You may freeze chicken casserole as a soothing and simple meal to make. Cooked spaghetti, canned veggies, and a sauce like Alfredo or tomato sauce are combined with cooked chicken to form this dish. After chilling, place in a freezer bag or airtight container.

It's crucial to label meals with the date and contents when preparing them to be frozen. Also, it's crucial to confirm that all substances are secure and suitable for the child's dietary requirements and allergies.

In conclusion, parents and other caregivers of children with cancer may find it useful to prepare meals in large quantities that may be frozen. Even on days when they may not feel like cooking or eating, parents can make sure their children have access to wholesome meals by employing a range of items and recipes.

Making soups and stews suitable for Children

While it might be hard to get youngsters enthused about soups and stews occasionally, they can be a healthy and soothing dinner choice for children with cancer. The following advice can help you make soups and stews more kid-friendly:

- Choose tasty and vibrant ingredients: Try adding a range of colorful veggies like carrots, sweet potatoes, and bell peppers to your soup or stew since kids like vivid colors and intriguing textures. Adding colorful shapes like little meatballs or alphabet spaghetti is another option.

- Make it straightforward: Youngsters often choose straightforward and well-known tastes, so don't be afraid to make your soup or stew simple. Using basic herbs and spices like salt, pepper, and parsley, try a traditional chicken noodle soup or a beef and vegetable stew.
- Create your toppings: Kids adore toppings, so let them add shredded cheese, croutons, or a dab of sour cream to their bowl of soup or stew. You may also experiment with using interesting and surprising toppings like tortilla strips or potato chip crumbs.
- Utilize a slow cooker: Soups and stews may be easily prepared with slow cookers. They also give the tastes more time to mix, making the food more tasty and delicate. Kids also like the anticipation of waking up to a stew that smells good.
- Serve with bread: Soup and stew go well with bread, and youngsters often like the chance to dip and dunk. To make your

soup or stew even more alluring, try serving it with warm crusty bread or buns.

- Make it enjoyable: Eating stew and soup may be messy and enjoyable. Consider serving your child's soup in amusing bowls or cups, or even allow them to use straws. This may give the dinner a fun and exciting quality.

You may increase your kids' enjoyment and attractiveness of soups and stews by using these suggestions. To determine what will benefit your kid the most, don't be afraid to experiment and be creative with the ingredients and presentation.

<u>Chapter 5</u>

<u>Major Dishes</u>

For children undergoing cancer treatment to maintain their general health and wellness, nutritious meals are essential. Here are some suggestions for major meals that are pleasant, simple, and nutritional for children with cancer:

- Roasted veggies with grilled chicken: Herbs and spices are a simple way to season the grilled chicken, which is a fantastic source of protein. Sweet potatoes, broccoli, and other roasted veggies may provide a range of nutrients and colors to the meal.
- The traditional meal of spaghetti with tomato sauce and meatballs is a favorite among young diners. Make your tomato sauce with fresh herbs and whole wheat pasta for additional nutrients and fiber. Ground beef or turkey may be used to

make meatballs, which can also be baked for a healthy choice.

- Fish is a wonderful source of omega-3 fatty acids and is simply cooked by baking or grilling. It goes well with quinoa and roasted veggies. Quinoa may be seasoned with herbs and spices to give it a taste, and it is a wonderful source of protein. Asparagus, zucchini, and bell peppers are a few examples of roasted veggies that may offer more nutrition and color to the meal.

- Stir-fried chicken with vegetables: This fast and simple recipe is nutrient-rich and can be made in a matter of minutes. Add low-sodium soy sauce, ginger, and garlic to make a tasty sauce, along with boneless chicken breast, and a variety of veggies such as bell peppers, carrots, and snow peas.

- Black beans, cheese, and salsa may be added to baked sweet potatoes for extra protein and taste. Baked sweet potatoes are a fantastic source of fiber. This meal is simple to make and may be altered to suit a child's culinary tastes.

- Meals should be made using fresh, high-quality ingredients, and processed foods that are heavy in sugar, salt, and bad fats should be avoided. Together with collaborating with a healthcare professional or registered dietitian, parents, and caregivers should take into account the child's specific dietary requirements and preferences to make sure they are obtaining the right nutrients while undergoing treatment.

Delicious easy-to-make dinners

Finding entrée ideas for meals that are not only wholesome and filling but also fast and simple to make may at times be difficult. Here are a few scrumptious and simple dinner recipes that are ideal for weeknights on the go or when you need a fast and filling supper.

- Chicken skewers that have been grilled simply need a few ingredients and may be made in 20 minutes. Chicken breast cubes should be marinated in olive oil, lemon juice, garlic, and your preferred herbs and spices before being skewered and cooked to perfection. For a full supper, serve with a side salad or grilled veggies.

- Salmon and veggies cooked in a single pan: This meal is not only nutritious but also easy to prepare and clean up. Place the salmon fillets and a variety of chopped veggies, including bell peppers, broccoli, and zucchini, on a sheet pan. Sprinkle with salt and pepper, drizzle with olive oil, and bake for 15 to 20 minutes. This dish is not only tasty but also loaded with vitamins, minerals, and omega-3 fatty acids.

- Kids and adults alike love this traditional meal of spaghetti with tomato sauce and meatballs. For more nutrition and fiber, use whole wheat spaghetti and homemade tomato sauce with fresh herbs. Ground beef or turkey may be used to make meatballs, which can also be baked for a healthy choice.

- This vegetarian dish, a wrap with vegetables and hummus, is ideal for people seeking a fast and wholesome supper choice. Spread hummus on a piece of whole wheat bread and top with a variety of finely chopped veggies, such as bell peppers, carrots, and cucumbers. Enjoy it rolled up!
- Black beans, cheese, and salsa may be added to baked sweet potatoes for extra protein and taste. Baked sweet potatoes are a fantastic source of fiber. This meal is simple to make and may be altered to suit your tastes.

It's crucial to include a range of nutrient-dense foods in dinners, including as lean protein, complete grains, and veggies. You can make sure you are obtaining the nutrients you need to maintain your general health and wellness by doing this. Also, these dishes are simple to adapt to your taste preferences and dietary requirements, adding to the fun and satisfaction of mealtime.

In conclusion, these mouthwatering and simple-to-prepare dinners are ideal for hectic weeknights or for times when you need a fast and filling supper. You can make sure you are receiving the nutrients you need to support your general health and wellness by consuming a range of nutrient-dense meals according to your taste preferences.

<u>Meat and vegetarian choices</u>

Suggestions for accompaniments and sides:
To meet various dietary preferences and constraints, it's crucial to take both vegetarian and meat-based choices into account when preparing meals. Here are some suggestions for meals that are both vegetarian and meat-based, along with the appropriate sides and toppings.

A.)Options for vegetarians:

- Quinoa and black bean salad: This vegetarian dish is a great option for a light lunch or supper since it's high in protein and fiber. Quinoa needs just to be cooked before being combined with black beans, diced tomatoes, and veggies like bell peppers.

- Stir-fried veggies: You may add your preferred vegetables and a protein source like tofu or tempeh to this simple recipe. Just add your protein source to a wok or pan of stir-fried veggies like broccoli, bell peppers, and carrots, along with a homemade sauce.

- Lentil soup: Packed with protein and fiber, this hearty soup is ideal for a chilly winter day. To enhance flavor, just cook lentils with veggies like carrots, celery, and onions along with your preferred herbs and spices.

B.)Options depending on meat:

- Chicken breast that has been grilled is a traditional dish that can be seasoned with herbs and spices and is a fantastic source of lean protein. Chicken breast should simply be marinated in olive oil with your preferred herbs and spices before being grilled till done.
- Beef stir-fry: For people who want a flavorful and filling supper, this recipe is ideal. Stir-fry beef simply with veggies like broccoli, bell peppers, and carrots while using a homemade sauce for flavor.
- Salmon baked in the oven is a filling and healthful main dish that is quick and simple to make. Salmon fillets should be

seasoned with your preferred herbs and spices before baking for 15-20 minutes.

C.)Accouterments and side dishes:
- Vegetables that have been roasted: Vegetables that have been roasted include broccoli, carrots, and cauliflower. These foods are tasty and healthful. Vegetables should just be tossed with olive oil, salt, and pepper before roasting for 20 to 30 minutes in the oven.
- Quinoa pilaf is a high-protein, high-fiber side dish that makes a wonderful substitution for regular rice pilaf. Quinoa may be prepared easily with vegetable broth and flavor-enhancing ingredients like sautéed onions and parsley and thyme.
- Garlic mashed potatoes are a traditional side dish that goes well with any dinner and are simple to make. Boil potatoes until fork-tender, then mash with butter and garlic. Add salt and pepper to taste.

To summarize, it's important to take varied dietary preferences and limits into account when preparing meals by taking both vegetarian and meat-based choices into account. You can make sure you are receiving the nutrients you need to support your general health and wellness by consuming a range of nutrient-dense meals according to your taste preferences. Moreover, side dishes and accompaniments may improve the taste and nutritional content of your entrée, adding to the satisfaction and enjoyment of meals.

Chapter 6

Sweets & Desserts: Cancer is a terrible condition for anybody to deal with, but it may be particularly difficult for kids. Loss of appetite, nausea and altered taste are just a few of the many side effects of cancer therapies that may make it challenging for children with cancer to enjoy food. Yet, giving children the nutrition and energy they need to combat cancer while also giving them something to look forward to throughout treatment, snacks, and desserts may be a terrific idea.There are several things to take into account when selecting sweets and desserts for children with cancer. First and foremost, it's critical to keep in mind that everyone facing cancer, even children, has to eat a nutritious, well-balanced diet. To do this, they must consume a lot of fruits, vegetables, whole grains, lean protein, and healthy fats. Desserts and sweets have to be seen as an addition to their regular meals rather than a substitute.

It's crucial to take into account the particular dietary demands and limits of children with cancer when selecting snacks and desserts for them. For instance, some kids may need to avoid certain foods that might hurt them because of a compromised immune system brought on by chemotherapy or radiation. Due to their cancer treatment, some kids could have certain dietary limitations, such as staying away from meals with a lot of sugar or fat.

Smoothies are a fantastic alternative to sweets and desserts for children with cancer. Smoothies may be made using nutrient-dense fruits and vegetables and can be altered to suit the nutritional requirements and tastes of each kid. For instance, adding a sweet fruit, like a banana, or honey might help cover up any bitter or metallic flavors if a youngster is experiencing taste alterations. To assist add more calories and protein to smoothies, nut kinds of butter or protein powder may be used.

Homemade popsicles are another alternative to sweets and desserts for children with cancer. Fruit juice, yogurt, or even pureed fruits and vegetables may be used to make these. A fun treat for kids to create themselves, homemade popsicles may be a terrific way to remain hydrated and give necessary vitamins and minerals.Children with cancer may still enjoy cookies and other baked goods, but it's crucial to choose recipes that are reduced in sugar and fat. These snacks may be made healthier by substituting honey or maple syrup for refined sugar and whole-grain flour for white flour to add additional fiber and nutrients to the dessert.

Moreover, it's important to keep in mind that snacks and desserts have other purposes than providing nutrients, such as providing solace and satisfaction. Treats and sweets may help children with cancer feel normal and live their lives to the fullest despite the difficulties they are experiencing. In addition to making sure that these delights are wholesome and nourishing, it's crucial to keep in mind that they should also be enjoyable, delectable, and something to look forward to.

Dessert recipes that are healthy and won't interfere with therapy

Chemotherapy and radiation therapy for cancer may significantly affect a person's appetite and taste preferences. Because of this, it may be challenging for those who are receiving treatment to consume the foods necessary to strengthen their immune systems and keep up their strength. A good method to provide cancer patients with the nutrition they need without interfering with their treatment is to create nutritious desserts that are suited to their unique dietary demands and limitations.

Here are some dessert recipes that are healthy and won't affect cancer treatment:

- An easy dessert that is nutrient-dense is baked apples with cinnamon and walnuts. Walnuts are a wonderful source of omega-3 fatty acids, while apples are abundant in fiber and antioxidants. Just core an apple and fill it with a combination of cinnamon, walnuts, and honey to create this treat. Bake in the oven for 20 to 30 minutes, or until the filling is golden and the apple is tender.

- Avocado Chocolate Mousse: Avocado is a nutrient-rich food that is rich in fiber and heart-healthy fats. Moreover, it has a moderate taste that makes it a fantastic foundation for a creamy dessert. Blend the ripe avocado, cocoa powder, honey, and a dash of vanilla essence until creamy to form the mousse. Serve chilled with whipped cream or fresh berries.
- Greek Yogurt Parfait: Greek yogurt is a fantastic choice for cancer patients who need to maintain their strength without ingesting too much sugar since it is rich in protein and low in sugar. Layer Greek yogurt, fresh fruit, almonds, and a drizzle of honey or maple syrup to create a parfait. To make this dish more fascinating, you may add various kinds of fruit and toppings.

- Chia Seed Pudding: Chia seeds are a fantastic source of protein, omega-3 fatty acids, and fiber. They take on a gel-like consistency after being soaked in liquid, which makes them an excellent pudding basis. Chia seeds, milk (dairy or non-dairy), honey or maple syrup, and vanilla extract are combined to produce chia seed pudding. Serve the mixture with fresh fruit or nuts after letting it chill in the fridge for at least two hours or overnight.

- Berry Sorbet: For cancer patients who need to restrict their consumption of dairy products, sorbet is an excellent substitute for ice cream. Blend frozen berries (such as raspberries, strawberries, or blueberries), honey or maple syrup, and a little bit of lemon juice to create berry sorbet. Either serve right now or freeze for later.

Cancer is a complicated condition that may impact a person's appetite, metabolism, and nutritional status

Nutrition and Cancer

For cancer patients, a healthy diet is crucial because it may strengthen their immune systems, keep them strong, and lower their risk of problems during treatment.

Following are a few crucial elements of a diet for cancer patients:

- Calories and protein: To maintain their weight and muscular mass, cancer patients often need more calories and protein than healthy people. This is because cancer cells may use a lot of the body's resources and energy. Some patients may need a high-calorie, high-protein diet depending on the stage of their cancer and the sort of therapy they are receiving. Lean meats, fish, poultry, eggs, dairy goods, beans, and nuts are all excellent sources of protein.

- Vitamins and minerals: Vitamins and minerals are crucial for the immune system and general health. Due to the strain of therapy and the disease's impact on the body, cancer patients may need more nutrients. A range of vitamins and minerals should be obtained through dietary sources such as fruits, vegetables, whole grains, and fortified goods. A licensed dietician can assist in determining nutritional requirements and, if required, offer the right supplements. Keeping hydrated is crucial for cancer patients to support healthy digestion, renal function, and general well-being. Dehydration may result from cancer treatments like chemotherapy and radiation, so it's crucial to consume enough fluids, particularly water. It's crucial to speak with a healthcare provider since certain cancer patients may need to restrict their fluid intake owing to specific medical concerns.

- Weight management: Cancer patients must maintain a healthy weight since both obesity and malnutrition may have a detrimental effect on how well they respond to therapy. To assist in maintaining a healthy weight, a licensed dietitian may assist in creating a tailored dietary plan.
- Dietary Restrictions: Depending on their medical condition or therapy, some cancer patients may need to avoid certain foods or nutrients. For instance, people who have mouth sores or trouble swallowing may need to steer clear of meals that are hot or acidic. It may be necessary to steer clear of meals that are crunchy or hard for patients receiving radiation treatment to the head and neck. Some dietary changes or medicines may be used to treat certain chemotherapy therapies' potential side effects of nausea and vomiting. The development of suitable meal plans and identification of any essential dietary restrictions should be done in

collaboration with a healthcare practitioner.

In conclusion, cancer sufferers must consume the right foods to support their therapy and preserve their health. The nutrients required for optimum health may be provided by a well-balanced diet that contains plenty of fruits, vegetables, whole grains, lean protein, and healthy fats. Making ensuring that dietary requirements are satisfied and any required limits are followed may be facilitated by working with a qualified dietitian or healthcare practitioner.

Nutritional issues during cancer therapy

For patients and their families, cancer treatment may be a trying and stressful period, and nutrition often suffers as a result. Yet, keeping a healthy diet during cancer treatment is crucial for boosting the immune system, minimizing side effects, and raising the general quality of life.

Following are some food concerns for cancer patients:

- Handling Side Effects: There are a variety of side effects that may result from cancer therapies like chemotherapy and radiation, including nausea, vomiting, diarrhea, constipation, mouth sores, and changes in appetite. Patients may find it difficult to eat and maintain a healthy diet as a result of these adverse effects. To manage these side effects and alter diet as necessary, it's crucial to see a qualified dietitian or another healthcare provider. For instance, people who are nauseated and vomiting may find it easier to handle short, frequent meals or bland foods.

- Addressing Calorie and Protein Needs: To maintain their weight and muscular mass, cancer patients often need more calories and protein than healthy people do. This is because cancer cells may use a lot of the body's resources and energy. Some patients may need a high-calorie, high-protein diet depending on the stage of their cancer and the sort of therapy they are receiving. Lean meats, fish, poultry, eggs, dairy goods, beans, and nuts are all excellent sources of protein.

- Appropriate Fluid Intake: Maintaining normal kidney function, digestion, and general health for cancer patients means staying hydrated. Dehydration may result from cancer treatments like chemotherapy and radiation, so it's crucial to consume enough fluids, particularly water. It's crucial to speak with a healthcare provider since certain cancer patients may need to restrict their fluid intake owing to specific medical concerns.
- Vitamin and mineral supplements may be necessary for certain cancer patients to assist them to satisfy their nutritional demands. This is particularly true for people who have trouble eating as a result of adverse effects from their treatments. A licensed dietitian or healthcare provider may assist in determining nutritional

requirements and provide suitable supplement recommendations.

- Dietary Restrictions: Depending on their medical condition or therapy, some cancer patients may need to avoid certain foods or nutrients. For instance, people who have mouth sores or trouble swallowing may need to steer clear of meals that are hot or acidic. It may be necessary to steer clear of meals that are crunchy or hard for patients receiving radiation treatment to the head and neck. Some dietary changes or medicines may be used to treat certain chemotherapy therapies' potential side effects of nausea and vomiting. The development of suitable meal plans and identification of any essential dietary restrictions should be done in collaboration with a healthcare practitioner.

There are several more crucial variables to bear in mind throughout cancer therapy in addition to the dietary issues already mentioned:

- Food safety: As a result of their medical treatments, cancer patients may have weaker immune systems, rendering them more vulnerable to foodborne infections. It's critical to adopt excellent food safety practices, such as washing hands before handling raw or undercooked meals and cooking meats to the proper temperatures. Patients should also stay away from deli meats that have been left out for a lengthy period and unpasteurized dairy products.
- Physical exercise is crucial for cancer patients undergoing treatment because it may boost mood, alleviate tiredness, and increase energy. Moreover, exercise may support bone and muscular density maintenance. Before beginning an exercise program, it's vital to speak with a healthcare provider since some individuals may need to restrict physical activity

based on their treatment and general health.

- Emotional Support: Patients undergoing cancer treatment may feel emotionally exhausted and may struggle with anxiety, sadness, or other mental health issues. At this period, patients should get emotional support, and if necessary, they should have access to therapy or other services. Patients must have a network of friends and relatives who can encourage them and assist with daily duties.
- Smoking and Drinking: Smoking and drinking may have a detrimental impact on the results of cancer treatments and general health. Smoking and excessive drinking should be avoided by cancer patients since they both raise the risk of complications and compromise the efficacy of therapy.

After receiving cancer treatment, patients must have follow-up care and monitoring to make sure the disease doesn't come back. This might be routine examinations, imaging testing, or other kinds of doctor's visits. Patients should keep their attention focused on keeping a healthy diet and general well-being.

In conclusion, cancer treatment necessitates a variety of dietary and lifestyle choices. To manage treatment-related side effects, maintain a healthy diet, and support overall health and well-being, patients must receive support and guidance from medical professionals, registered dietitians, and support systems.

Foods to stay away from During Cancer Treatments.

Cancer treatments may be difficult and can have a variety of side effects that might affect a patient's appetite, taste, and digestion. Patients must keep a nutritious diet throughout this period since it promotes their general well-being and aids in the management of treatment-related side effects. Avoiding some foods that may worsen side effects or interfere with the efficacy of therapy may be a part of eating a balanced diet. Following are some meals to steer clear of when battling cancer:

- Meals that are uncooked or raw may raise the risk of foodborne diseases, which can be particularly risky for cancer patients with compromised immune systems. Uncooked or raw foods include meat, chicken, fish, and eggs. Avoiding raw or undercooked meals can help to lower the risk of illness. Cook meats and eggs to the proper temperature.
- Unpasteurized Dairy Products: During cancer treatment, patients should avoid unpasteurized dairy products including raw milk and soft cheeses since they increase the risk of contracting foodborne diseases. Dairy products that have been pasteurized may be a healthy source of calcium and protein and are safe to eat.
- Hot or Acidic Foods: Spicy or acidic meals may irritate the digestive tract and increase symptoms like nausea, vomiting, and heartburn. Examples include hot peppers, citrus fruits, and tomatoes.

Patients should avoid these items or consume them in moderation while receiving cancer therapy.

- Fried or fatty meals may be hard to digest and can result in diarrhea or other digestive problems. Examples include fast food, processed snacks, and high-fat meats. Patients should try to eat healthy fats from foods like avocados, nuts, seeds, and fatty seafood.

- Meals high in sugar may promote blood sugar increases and weight gain, which can be dangerous for cancer patients. Foods high in sugar include candy, cookies, and soda. Patients should eat carbs from whole grains, fruits, and vegetables as well as other nutritious foods.

- Alcohol: As it might reduce the efficiency of cancer treatments, it should be avoided while receiving them. Moreover, alcohol may make symptoms like nausea, vomiting, and dehydration worse.

- Certain fruits and vegetables: Some fruits and vegetables might conflict with some cancer treatment regimens. For instance, cruciferous foods like broccoli and kale may interfere with thyroid function in people undergoing certain therapies, while grapefruit and its juice may interact with certain chemotherapy medications. A healthcare expert should be consulted to see if any food restrictions are required depending on specific treatment plans.

Following a healthy diet while receiving treatment:

Children with cancer should maintain a balanced diet because it helps promote general health and well-being, control adverse effects from therapy, and enhance treatment success. Children may find it difficult to maintain a balanced diet throughout cancer treatment, however, since their appetite, taste, and digestion may alter. Here are some pointers for keeping up a healthy diet when a kid is receiving cancer treatment:

- Provide Nutrient-Dense Foods: Children with cancer should eat nutrient-dense meals including fruits, vegetables, whole grains, and lean meats because they contain vital nutrients that promote overall health and well-being. Provide them with a choice of vibrant fruits and veggies, whole grain loaves of bread and cereals, lean meats, fish, and chicken, as well as low-fat dairy items.

- Urge Kids to Eat Little, Frequently: Children with cancer may suffer changes in appetite and may not feel like eating big meals. It might be easier to make sure they are receiving enough calories and nutrients if you encourage them to eat small, frequent meals and snacks throughout the day.

- Make Meals Appetizing: A kid receiving cancer treatment may experience changes in taste or become more sensitive to specific tastes or textures. Using seasonings, herbs, and spices to improve taste and food presentation to make food more aesthetically pleasing, it's crucial to make meals and snacks as attractive as possible.

- Texture modifications should be taken into consideration since certain cancer therapies might make it difficult for kids to swallow or digest certain meals. Consider changing the food's texture if a youngster is having trouble with a certain texture, such as by pureeing or mixing fruits and vegetables.
- Keep Hydrated: Kids with cancer must keep hydrated during treatment since dehydration may make side symptoms like exhaustion, nausea, and constipation worse. During the day, provide lots of fluids, such as water, juice, milk, and soups.

A child's ability to eat and absorb nutrients might be negatively impacted by side effects from several cancer therapies, such as nausea, vomiting, and diarrhea. Develop a meal plan that takes into account any dietary limitations or changes in appetite while collaborating with a healthcare practitioner to control side effects.

Children should be included in the meal planning process since it may make them feel more invested in their care and be both a fun and instructive activity. When appropriate, encourage kids to participate in meal planning, grocery shopping, and food preparation.

In conclusion, it's critical for children receiving cancer therapy to maintain a nutritious diet. Parents and caregivers can support children's overall health and well-being during this trying time by providing nutrient-dense foods, encouraging small, frequent meals, making meals appealing, modifying textures if necessary, staying hydrated, being aware of side effects, and involving children in meal planning. To make sure that their child's dietary requirements are being addressed, it is advised that families engage closely with their medical team.

<u>Chapter 7</u>

<u>Resources to Explore</u>

Families may feel overwhelmed by a child's cancer diagnosis, and it may be difficult to know where to turn for advice and support. The following materials may be useful for families:

- The American Childhood Cancer Organization (ACCO) is a nonprofit organization whose goal is to make life better for families with cancer-stricken children. They provide details and resources on a range of issues relating to pediatric cancer, such as available treatments, financial aid, and support services.

- National Cancer Institute (NCI): The NCI is an organization of the government that offers thorough information about cancer, particularly pediatric cancer. Their website offers information about clinical studies, diagnostics, and support services.

- Children's Oncology Group (COG): COG is the biggest organization in the world devoted to research into pediatric cancer and offers assistance and support to parents of children with the disease. Their website offers information about available therapies, medical studies, and supportive care.
- CancerCare: Children and their families are welcome to receive free professional support services from CancerCare, a national nonprofit organization. They provide options for education, financial aid, and counseling.Families of children who are undergoing treatment at a hospital distance from their home may stay in a temporary residence thanks to Ronald McDonald House Charities (RMHC). They have sites throughout the country and provide families with a place to stay when things are tough.
- Leading children's hospital St. Jude is dedicated to treating and curing conditions that are life-threatening for children, such

as cancer. They provide therapy, palliative care, and research to kids and their families in addition to comprehensive care.

During a health crisis, a family may use the free websites provided by the nonprofit group CaringBridge to exchange information and stay in touch with one another. It may be a useful tool to educate loved ones, foster a feeling of community, and provide support.Families may get help from these sources as well as their medical staff, social workers, and neighborhood cancer support groups. Families need to know they are not alone and that there are numerous options available to them to assist them get through this trying time.

Resources for Financial Assistance

- The National Cancer Institute provides a listing of businesses that help cancer sufferers financially:

https://www.cancer.gov/about-cancer/managing-care/track-care-costs/financial-help-resources

- A nationwide nonprofit organization called CancerCare provides financial aid, counseling, and other forms of support to those impacted by cancer: https://www.cancercare.org/
- The American Cancer Society provides many financial aid programs, including help with hotel and transportation: https://www.cancer.org/treatment/support-programs-and-services/patient-lodging/hope-lodge.html
- Financial aid is available through the Leukemia & Lymphoma Society for co-payments, insurance premiums, and travel expenses: https://www.lls.org/support/financial-support

Services for counseling and support groups:

- For families of children with cancer, The Children's Oncology Group provides a range of information and support services, such as counseling and support groups: https://childrensoncologygroup.org/index.php/survivorship-resources/for-families/
- For families of children with cancer, the National Cancer Institute offers a list of support organizations: https://www.cancer.gov/types/childhood-cancers/patient/childhood-support
- The American Cancer Society provides a range of support services, such as cancer helplines and online support groups: https://www.cancer.org/treatment/support-programs-and-services.html
- For families impacted by cancer, CancerCare offers counseling services, as well as support groups for parents and siblings of cancer-stricken children: https://www.cancercare.org/individuals-families/children-teens-and-young-adults-with-cancer

In conclusion, this cookbook for children with cancer is an important tool for families who are struggling with this disease. It not only offers wholesome and delectable dishes for kids receiving cancer treatment, but it may also strengthen family ties and create happy memories in the kitchen. This cookbook may support kids in keeping their strength and energy levels during their treatment by using items that are healthful and simple to digest. Also, it might provide children with a feeling of normality at a time when their lives are often upended by hospital stays and medical procedures. Overall, this book has the potential to be a helpful and inspiring resource that equips families to assist their child's recovery process.

www.ingramcontent.com/pod-product-compliance
Lightning Source LLC
Chambersburg PA
CBHW050808250726
48653CB00006B/2133